MW00908473

Junior Drug Awareness

Marijuana

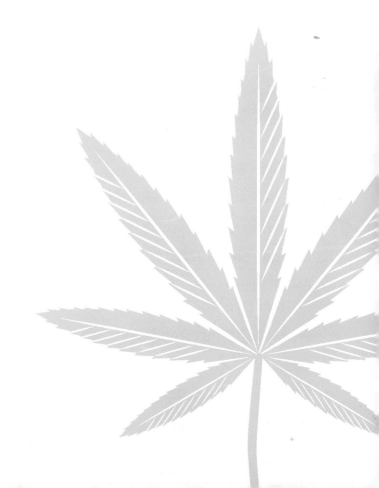

Junior Drug Awareness

Junior Drug Awareness

Marijuana

Introduction by **BARRY R. McCAFFREY**
Director, Office of National Drug Control Policy

Foreword by **STEVEN L. JAFFE, M.D.**
Professor of Child and Adolescent Psychiatry,
Emory University

Judy L. Hasday, Ed.M.
Therese De Angelis

Chelsea House Publishers
Philadelphia

To the kids—Tiffany, Elyse, Adam, Ben, and Aaron—who are always a source of joy for me.
With love, Aunt Judy   —JLH

To Rich, Marie, Joe, Bernadette, Elizabeth, Christine, and Audrey. May you live long, happy,
and healthy lives. Love, Aunt Therese   —TD

CHELSEA HOUSE PUBLISHERS
Editor in Chief Stephen Reginald
Production Manager Pamela Loos
Director of Photography Judy L. Hasday
Art Director Sara Davis
Managing Editor James D. Gallagher
Senior Production Editor Lisa Chippendale

Staff for MARIJUANA
Senior Editor Therese De Angelis
Associate Art Director/Designer Takeshi Takahashi
Picture Researcher Patricia Burns
Cover Illustrator/Designer Takeshi Takahashi

Cover photo © 1997 Charles Gupton/The Stock Market

http://www.chelseahouse.com

3 5 7 9 8 6 4

Library of Congress Cataloging-in-Publication Data
Hasday, Judy L., 1957-
Marijuana. Judy L. Hasday, Therese De Angelis; intro-
duction by Barry R. McCaffrey; Steven L. Jaffe, consult-
ing editor.
80 pp.   cm. — (Junior drug awareness)
Includes bibliographical references and index.
Summary: Describes the nature and effects of marijua-
na, why people use it, and the dangers of its use.
ISBN 0-7910-5176-5 (hardcover)
1. Marijuana—Juvenile literature. 2. Drug abuse—Juve-
nile literature. [1. Marijuana. 2. Drug abuse.] I. De
Angelis, Therese. II. Jaffe, Steven L., 1940- . III. Title.
IV. Series.
HV5822.M3H37 1998
362.29'5—dc21   98-51362
                                                            CIP
                                                            AC

CONTENTS

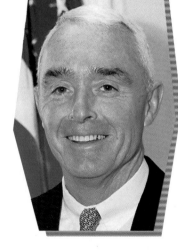

by **Barry R. McCaffrey**
Director, Office of National
Drug Control Policy

STAYING AWAY FROM ILLEGAL DRUGS, TOBACCO PRODUCTS, AND ALCOHOL

G ood health allows you to be as strong, happy, smart, and skillful as you can possibly be. The worst thing about illegal drugs is that they damage people from the inside. Our bodies and minds are wonderful, complicated systems that run like finely tuned machines when we take care of ourselves.

Doctors prescribe legal drugs, called medicines, to heal us when we become sick, but dangerous chemicals that are not recommended by doctors, nurses, or pharmacists are called illegal drugs. These drugs cannot be bought in stores because they harm different organs of the body, causing illness or even death. Illegal drugs, such as marijuana, cocaine or "crack," heroin, metham-phetamine ("meth"), and other dangerous substances are against the law because they affect our ability to think, work, play, sleep, or eat.

If anyone ever offers you illegal drugs or any kind of pills, liquids, substances to smoke, or shots to inject into your body, tell them you're not interested. You should report drug pushers—people who distribute these poisons—to parents, teachers, police, coaches, clergy, or other adults whom you trust.

Cigarettes and alcohol are also illegal for youngsters. Tobacco products and drinks like wine, beer, and liquor are particularly harmful for children and teenagers because their bodies, especially their nervous systems, are still developing. For this reason, young people are more likely to be hurt by illicit drugs—including cigarettes and alcohol. These two products kill more people—from cancer, and automobile accidents caused by intoxicated drivers—than all other drugs combined. We say about drug use: "Users are losers." Be a winner and stay away from illegal drugs, tobacco products, and alcoholic beverages.

Here are four reasons why you shouldn't use illegal drugs:

- Illegal drugs can cause brain damage.
- Illegal drugs are "psychoactive." This means that they change your personality or the way you feel. They also impair your judgment. While under the influence of drugs, you are more likely to endanger your life or someone else's. You will also be less able to protect yourself from danger.
- Many illegal drugs are addictive, which means that once a person starts taking them, stopping is extremely difficult. An addict's body craves the drug and becomes dependent upon it. The illegal drug–user may become sick if the drug is discontinued and so may become a slave to drugs.

- Some drugs, called "gateway" substances, can lead a person to take more-dangerous drugs. For example, a 12-year-old who smokes marijuana is 79 times more likely to have an addiction problem later in life than a child who never tries marijuana.

Here are some reasons why you shouldn't drink alcoholic beverages, including beer and wine coolers:

- Alcohol is the second leading cause of death in our country. More than 100,000 people die every year because of drinking.
- Adolescents are twice as likely as adults to be involved in fatal alcohol-related car crashes.
- Half of all assaults against girls or women involve alcohol.
- Drinking is illegal if you are under the age of 21. You could be arrested for this crime.

Here are three reasons why you shouldn't smoke cigarettes:

- Nicotine is highly addictive. Once you start smoking, it is very hard to stop, and smoking cigarettes causes lung cancer and other diseases. Tobacco- and nicotine-related diseases kill more than 400,000 people every year.
- Each day, 3,000 kids begin smoking. One-third of these youngsters will probably have their lives shortened because of tobacco use.
- Children who smoke cigarettes are almost six times more likely to use other illegal drugs than kids who don't smoke.

If your parents haven't told you how they feel about the dangers of illegal drugs, ask them. One of every 10 kids aged 12 to 17 are using illegal drugs. They do not understand the risks they are taking with their health and their lives. However, the vast majority of young people in America are smart enough to figure out that drugs, cigarettes, and alcohol could rob them of their future. Be your body's best friend: guard your mental and physical health by staying away from drugs.

WHY SHOULD I LEARN ABOUT DRUGS?

Steven L. Jaffe, M.D.
Professor of Child and Adolescent Psychiatry, Emory University

Your grandparents and great-grandparents did not think much about "drug awareness." That's because drugs, to most of them, simply meant "medicine."

Of the three types of drugs, medicine is the good type. Medicines such as penicillin and aspirin promote healing and help sick people get better.

Another type of drug is obviously bad for you because it is poison. Then there are the kind of drugs that fool you, such as marijuana and LSD. They make you feel good, but they harm your body and brain.

Our great crisis today is that this third category of drugs has become widely abused. Drugs of abuse are everywhere, not just in rough neighborhoods. Many teens are introduced to drugs by older brothers, sisters, friends, or even friends' parents. Some people may use only a little bit of a drug, but others who inherited a tendency to become addicted may move on to using drugs all the time. If a family member is or was an alcoholic or an addict, a young person is at greater risk of becoming one.

Drug abuse can weaken us physically. Worse, it can cause permanent mental damage. Our brain is the most important part of our body. Our thoughts, hopes, wishes, feelings, and memories are located there, within 100 billion nerve cells. Alcohol and drugs that are abused will harm—and even destroy—these cells. During the teen years, your brain continues to develop and grow, but drugs and alcohol can impair this growth.

I treat all types of teenagers at my hospital programs and in my office. Many suffer from depression or anxiety. A lot of them abuse drugs and alcohol, and this makes their depression or fears worse. I have celebrated birthdays and high school graduations with many of my patients. But I have also been to sad funerals for others who have died from problems with drug abuse.

Doctors understand more about drugs today than ever before. We've learned that some substances (even some foods) that we once thought were harmless can actually cause health problems. And for some people, medicines that help relieve one symptom might cause problems in other ways. This is because each person's body chemistry and immune system are different.

For all of these reasons, drug awareness is important for everyone. We need to learn which drugs to avoid or question—not only the destructive, illegal drugs we hear so much about in the news, but also ordinary medicines we buy at the supermarket or pharmacy. We need to understand that even "good" drugs can hurt us if they are not used correctly. If we take any drug without a doctor's advice, we are taking a risk.

Drug awareness enables you to make good decisions. It allows you to become powerful and strong and have a meaningful life!

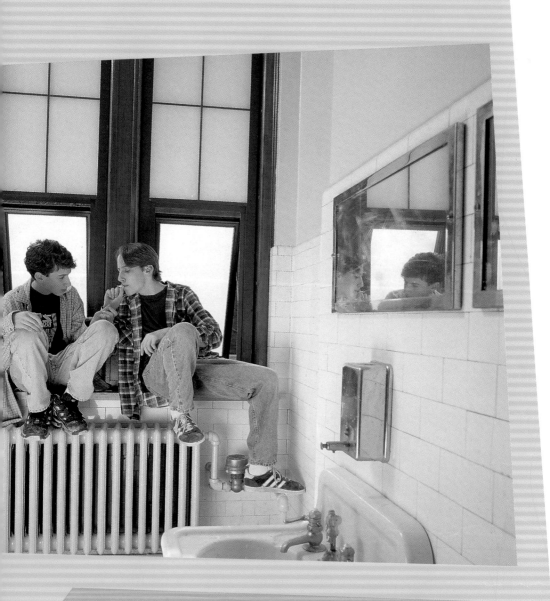

Smoking marijuana may seem harmless, but it can mess up your life. Your performance in school, sports, and other activities will suffer if you're high.

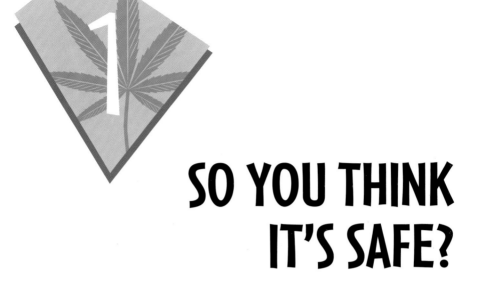

SO YOU THINK IT'S SAFE?

*I can still remember the first time I got high after smoking a marijuana **joint**. Although I was with friends, I wasn't comfortable with the new and strange sensations, and I became a little anxious. It didn't last long, however. My uneasiness began to fade away and was replaced by a mellow, relaxed state. I felt as though I had no worries and no pressures. Time seemed to slow to a crawl. My friends also seemed relaxed, slumped in chairs or on the couch, just hanging out like me, as music played in the background. We all seemed caught up in our own separate worlds.*

Most of my highs after that were a lot like that first one. Sometimes I felt giddy, and would laugh uncontrollably. Often I became extremely hungry, so I would devour butter almond ice cream or a box of dry frosted flakes. Then I would usually become drowsy and drift off to sleep. When I was awake, though, all of my senses seemed heightened. Colors were more vivid; music sounded better; food tasted incredible; and jokes were not just funny, they were hilarious. This drug was great. No hangovers, no aftereffects, no danger.

*I went on believing that until the day I got high at school. Up until then, I had always been pretty careful; after all, marijuana is illegal. Usually I only got high with my friends, but that day some of the people in the group were unfamiliar to me. A guy named Art had a **bong** that was so big it looked like a bassoon. There we all were, smoking someone's stash of marijuana with this very visible bong while sitting on the front lawn of the school. I remember thinking what a beautiful spring day it was. Not "Am I going to get caught? Will one of my teachers walk by? Will a cop drive by and see us all huddled around this pipe inhaling our lungs out?" I didn't want to get paranoid— that would have been no fun at all. Instead, I felt exhilarated at the risk I was taking.*

After a few minutes, though, I suddenly started to feel strange. My mouth became dry, and patches of blackness interfered with my vision. Voices became muffled and people's words sounded garbled. I broke out in a sweat. I was afraid I was going to be sick or pass out. My only thought was that I couldn't faint in front of my friends, so I got up and tried to get to my car, which was parked across the street. I figured if I was going to pass out, my car was the safest place to do it.

The thing is, I never made it there. In fact, I'm lucky I wasn't killed. When I stepped off the curb, feeling wobbly and disoriented, I didn't see the lunch truck coming down the street in my direction. Luckily, another student did, and he pushed me out of the way in time.

—Taylor, 16

You may think smoking marijuana is no big deal and poses no real danger. . . .

But did you know that using marijuana slows your reflexes and affects your timing and coordination? When you're high on marijuana, you may have trouble judging distances, and your reactions to sights and sounds are delayed. This might not sound dangerous to you, but what if your job required that you operate heavy equipment or make exact measurements? What if you had a job on a dangerous work site—like an aircraft carrier—and your coworkers were stoned?

On the evening of May 26, 1981, the USS *Nimitz,* which had been at sea for 11 days, moved quietly through the ocean off the coast of Florida. The calm was abruptly and violently shattered when a Navy jet attempting to land on the carrier slammed into the deck, hitting several fueled and armed F-14 fighter planes. Fuel tanks and ammunition exploded. The F-14s were ripped apart, and a missile on one of them ignited, creating a blazing inferno aboard the ship. By the following morning, 14 sailors were dead and 44 had been seriously injured. Twenty planes were damaged, at a cost of more than $100 million. Autopsies of the dead crew members revealed that six of them had traces of marijuana in their blood and urine.

You may think that smoking marijuana relaxes you and that it is a safe, "feel-good" drug. . . .

But did you know that using marijuana can cause short-term memory loss and distort your sense of time? Did you know that it can diminish your ability to perform mental and physical tasks?

On Sunday, January 4, 1987, at about 12:30 P.M., the Amtrak train *Colonial* pulled out of Union Station in Washington, D.C., with more than 600 passengers aboard. The train's final destination was Springfield, Massachusetts, about 800 miles north. It never got there.

At about 1:30 P.M., just a few minutes after a scheduled stop in Baltimore, Maryland, the *Colonial,* which was traveling at more than 100 miles an hour, collided with three Conrail diesel engines. The crash destroyed the Amtrak train's two electric locomotives, overturned its first five coaches, and derailed the seven passenger cars behind them. Early on Monday morning, hundreds of rescue workers assembled in the wake of the disaster were still searching among the mass of twisted metal for survivors and for the bodies of those who had died. In all, 16 passengers were killed and more than 170 were injured in one of the worst railroad accidents in history.

During the investigation into the crash, the Amtrak and Conrail employees involved in the disaster underwent blood and urine tests for the presence of drugs. The tests revealed that Conrail engineer Rick L. Gates and brakeman Edward Cromwell both had marijuana in

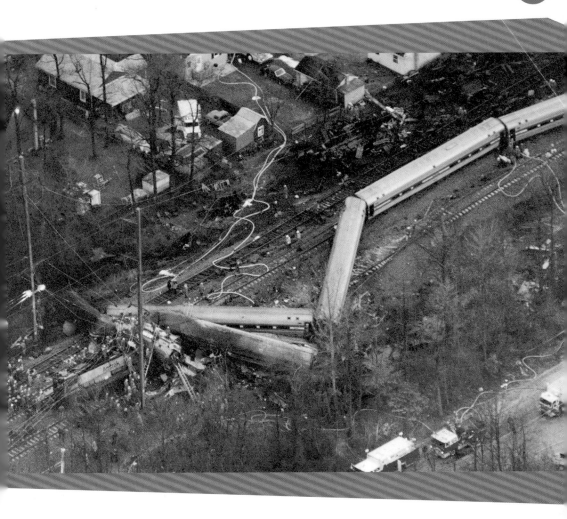

A photo of the derailed Amtrak passenger train in which 16 people were killed and 170 were injured in 1987. Drug tests showed that the engineer of the Conrail train that collided with this train had marijuana in his system.

their systems. Criminal charges were filed against Gates. Prosecutors believed that his use of marijuana had caused him to miss the stop signals meant to warn him of the approaching Amtrak train. Gates pleaded guilty to manslaughter but received only five years in prison.

You may think that you can smoke marijuana without wanting to try other drugs. . . .

But did you know that marijuana is a **gateway drug**—meaning that strong evidence shows that using marijuana leads to taking more powerful (and often lethal) drugs?

Although fans of famed *Saturday Night Live* comedian and actor John Belushi may not have known about his deadly drug habit, his friends and family did. In 1979, while Belushi was working on the film *The Blues Brothers,* he asked the doctor on the set, Bennett Braun, to give him a vitamin B-12 shot. Braun could see that the 30-year-old actor was abusing drugs. Belushi was overweight, his eyes were bloodshot, his skin was grayish, and his breathing was wheezy. Dr. Braun told Robert Weiss, the film's producer, "You've got to get him off drugs. . . . If you don't, get as many movies out of him as possible, because he has only two to three years to live."

On March 5, 1982, John Belushi was found dead of a drug overdose in his rented bungalow at the Chateau Marmont hotel in Hollywood, California. He had been **speed-**

Did You Know?

Like alcohol and cigarettes, marijuana is a "gateway" drug, which means that using it can lead to using more dangerous drugs. Sixty percent of kids who smoke pot before age 15 move on to cocaine. Kids aged 12 to 17 who smoke pot are 85 times more likely to use cocaine than those who do not smoke pot.

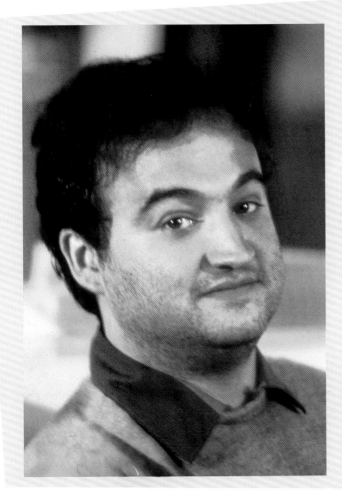

One of the many celebrities whose lives were cut short by drug abuse is John Belushi, who rose to fame as one of the early members of *Saturday Night Live.*

balling (injecting a mixture of cocaine and **heroin**).

John Belushi began using marijuana the summer after he graduated from high school. Over the next 16 years, Belushi abused many other drugs, including speed (a stimulant that increases the body's activity), **LSD,** and heroin. Many people who end up addicted to drugs have started out the same way—they begin smoking cigarettes or drinking beer or wine when they're young. Those who do are more likely to go on to using drugs that are more dangerous. And most people usually don't give up the drugs they began with. Instead, they add other chemicals to the harmful ones they're already using.

Unfortunately, John Belushi's untimely death from drug abuse is only one among thousands that occur each year. Stories such as his don't happen only to celebrities. Knowns and unknowns, athletes, politicians, businessmen, housewives, and kids all become victims of drug abuse. It can kill, and it often ruins careers, relationships, and lives.

Academy Award–winner Whoopi Goldberg also started smoking pot when she was a young girl. She began using LSD and other drugs not long after. Her drug abuse led her to drop out of high school and disappear from her community. When she was 17, she realized that she needed help, and she checked herself into a drug treatment program. Today she says, "There ain't no joy in a high—*none*. . . . You *think* there's a joy in a high because it feels good temporarily. But it feels good less and less often, so you've got to do it more and more often. . . . It ain't your friend. . . . I tell kids, 'save the money and just kill yourself because [if you're using drugs] that's what you're doing.'"

What Happened to Taylor?

I must have passed out after I was pushed out of the way of the lunch truck, because the next thing I remember was that I was flat on my back, looking up at the concerned faces of my friends.

I didn't know what happened. Just smoking **grass**

*wasn't supposed to do this to you. A thousand questions raced through my mind. Was the pot **laced** with some other drug? How could I be sure I wouldn't end up buying or smoking **tainted** pot again? Was it possible that, like other drugs, you could use marijuana several times and be fine, but then without warning get violently ill? Could that happen with a drug that was supposed to be so harmless? Had I done permanent damage to my health? If I couldn't be sure that smoking pot was safe, how could I be sure that I wouldn't become dependent on it or want to move on to other drugs?*

The answer was, I couldn't be sure of anything.

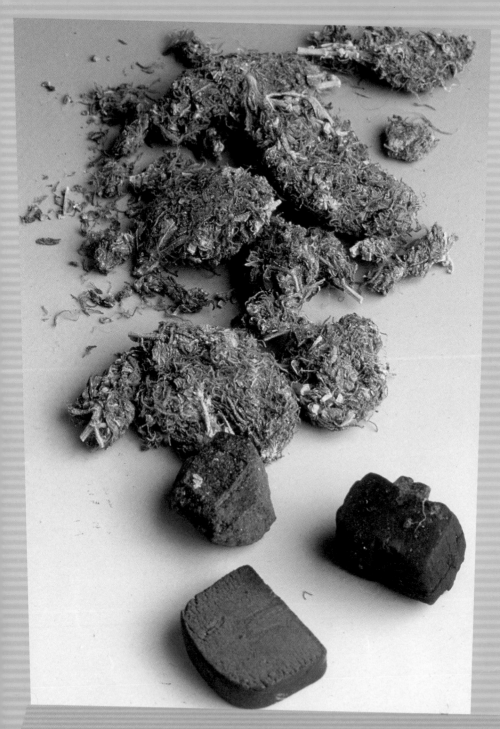

This photograph shows the drug products of the *Cannabis sativa* plant. At the top of the photo are dried leaves and flowering tops of the plant. At the bottom of the photo are several blocks of hashish, made by boiling the plant and filtering out solid particles, then letting the remaining substance cool and thicken.

WHAT IS MARIJUANA?

arijuana is the most frequently used illegal drug in America, and its popularity among adolescents is growing every day. According to the National Institutes of Health (NIH), marijuana use among eighth graders doubled between 1992 and 1995. Tenth and twelfth graders also showed increased marijuana use during these years. Recent surveys report that about one-third of high school seniors in the United States have tried marijuana at least once, and about 5 percent use the drug daily.

In addition, marijuana use has increased 38 percent among high school seniors in recent years. The number of seniors who believe that marijuana is harmful dropped by 22 percent between 1992 and 1995.

Why has this happened? Many factors are involved. One is that young people are seeing and hearing more pro-drug messages in the media, especially in the lyrics of the music they listen to. Even some clothing and accessories advertise the use of drugs. As a result, the misperception grows among both teens and adults that marijuana is a harmless **recreational** drug.

Where Does Marijuana Come From?

"Pot," "reefer," "grass," "weed," "Mary Jane," "herb," "gangsta," "skunk," "ganja"—there are more than 200 slang terms for marijuana, the green, brown, or gray mixture of dried, shredded flowers and leaves of the plant known as *Cannabis sativa.*

Sinsemilla, hashish, and **hashish oil** are more potent forms of marijuana. Sinsemilla (the word means "seedless") is produced from the unfertilized female cannabis plant. Hashish is made by boiling crushed marijuana leaves and stems in water to extract a sticky substance called **resin.** When cooled, the resin becomes a semisolid mass. The strongest form of cannabis, hashish oil, is produced with solvents like alcohol or gasoline. The finished product looks like a dark, gooey syrup, and it is 20 to 30 percent more powerful than other cannabis products.

Lots of people know how marijuana makes you feel, but did you know that the cannabis plant contains more than 400 chemicals? Several of them are **psychoactive,** which means that they can alter or change your brain. The chemical with the strongest effect on the brain is **THC (delta-9 tetrahydrocannabinol),** which is found in the resin of the plant. THC levels are the highest in the flower of the cannabis plant, which holds the highest concentration of resin.

How Do People Use Marijuana?

Dried marijuana leaves are usually rolled up in smoking papers and lit, much like the tobacco in a cigarette. The user tries to hold marijuana smoke in the lungs for as long as possible, so that its effects will be stronger.

In recent years, marijuana users have also begun making even bigger (and therefore more powerful) joints by filling emptied cigar wrappers with marijuana to make a **blunt.** The marijuana in blunts, like that in regular joints, is often mixed with other dangerous drugs or substances, such as cocaine, **PCP** (a synthetic painkiller known to cause violent behavior), and even embalming fluid (used to preserve corpses). Street names for these combinations include "primos," "oolies," "woolies," "happy sticks," "wicky sticks," "illies," and "shermans."

Marijuana smoke is also inhaled using pipes. Some pipes, called bongs, use water to cool the hot smoke before the user inhales it. Bongs also concentrate the smoke inside a chamber, so that it does not escape into the air.

A bong is one of many pieces of "equipment" used to prepare or inhale marijuana. These objects, called drug **paraphernalia,** also include **roach clips** and stones, which are used to hold the marijuana cigarette when it has burned down to a stub, and strainers to "clean" pot by separating twigs, seeds, and stems from the crushed leaves.

Another way people use marijuana is by ingesting it, by adding it to baked goods such as brownies or mixing it with beverages such as tea. Because the THC in "spiked" food and drinks goes to the user's stomach instead of the lungs, it takes longer to feel the effects of the drug. The high is not as intense as when marijuana is smoked, but it usually lasts longer.

How Long Has Marijuana Been Around?

The cannabis plant is one of the oldest known plants in the world, and it has had a variety of uses. The first known accounts of cannabis farming come from the Yang-shao culture of China in about 4500 B.C. These people harvested cannabis plants to make **hemp.** In a process known as **retting,** they soaked the rotted stems of the plants to loosen and separate the fibers, which were then fashioned into rope and netting.

Other ancient civilizations used the cannabis plant for medicinal, religious, and recreational purposes. The earliest known book about drugs, chemicals, and medicinal preparations, called the *Pên-ts'ao Ching,* described how cannabis helped ease painful ailments such as rheumatism, cramps, and constipation. It also made note of the psychoactive effects of the drug. Cultures in the Middle East and Europe learned of these qualities, and the use of cannabis spread to those regions.

Some historians believe that Native Americans were already using cannabis by the time European explorers

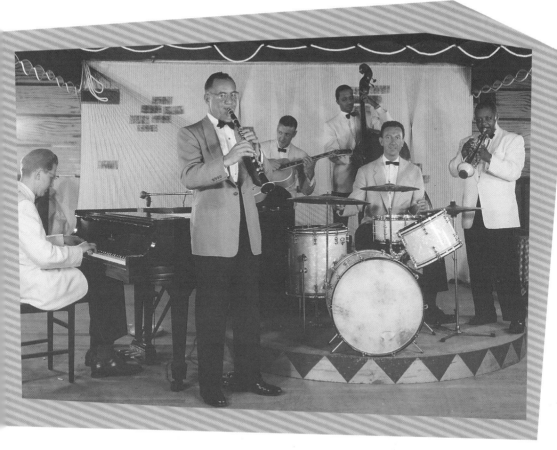

When your parents and grandparents were young, scientists and doctors had not yet learned about the harmful effects of marijuana. Many musicians believed that the drug made them more creative. Some, like bandleader Benny Goodman (shown here in 1954 with his orchestra), performed songs whose lyrics referred to marijuana.

arrived in the 16th century, although the explorers who settled in North America probably introduced the plant. The Europeans planted cannabis in the New World so that they would have a steady supply of hemp fiber to make rope and canvas sails for their ships. (Did you know that the word "canvas" is actually derived from the word "cannabis"?) As time passed, the products of the cannabis plant became so important that colonists in the early 18th century were required by law to grow it. American patriots like George Washington and Thomas Jefferson harvested cannabis crops on their own plantations.

Is Marijuana Beneficial or Dangerous?

During the mid-19th century, cannabis became popular for medical purposes. Researchers had discovered that preparations made from the cannabis plant were helpful in treating health problems such as headaches, insomnia (inability to sleep), and loss of appetite. In the beginning of the 20th century, it was legal for drugstores to carry medicines that contained marijuana.

By 1875, Americans had also discovered the practice of smoking marijuana and hashish for recreation. The custom was introduced in the Southwest by Mexican and Caribbean laborers and in eastern cities by Turkish merchants. From these areas, it spread across the country. Hashish parlors, where people gathered to smoke the drug, opened up in cities like New York and Chicago.

During the 1920s, marijuana use became popular among artists and musicians, many of whom believed that it enhanced their creativity. Jazz musician Fats Waller, for example, recorded a tune called "Reefer Song" that praised the virtues of the drug. Bandleader Benny Goodman's "Texas Tea Party" was another of many songs of that era that made reference to marijuana.

By the late 1920s, however, the public's concern over

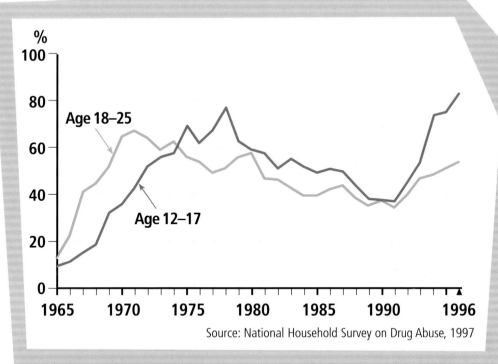

Source: National Household Survey on Drug Abuse, 1997

This graph, which covers the years 1965 to 1996, shows the percentage of people aged 12 to 17 and aged 18 to 25 who tried marijuana for the first time for each year represented. Look at the percentage of 12- to 17-year-olds who first tried marijuana in 1965 (lower left). The number is about 10 percent. Now look at the percentage of kids in that age group who first tried marijuana in the late 1970s. The number is almost 80 percent. The highest percentage of kids aged 12 to 17 years old who first tried marijuana was in 1996—more than 80 percent (upper right). Read Chapters 2 and 4 for some reasons why this happened.

the dangers of marijuana began to grow. A 1936 film called *Reefer Madness* was part of a widespread anti-marijuana campaign on the part of the media and the U.S. government. The information in the film, like much of the news about the drug that spread across the country, was so exaggerated that it seems comical to us today. At the same time, fear and hatred of blacks and immigrants, who were among the first recreational users, fueled a demand for laws that would make the drug illegal. States began passing their own laws to regulate marijuana, even though the plant was still being processed to make rope, paper, and fabric. The public began to associate marijuana with violent, wild, and uninhibited behavior.

In 1937, the U.S. Congress passed the Marijuana Tax Act, which heavily taxed manufacturers, importers, pharmacists, physicians, and anyone else who used, prescribed, or sold marijuana. Although the act did not actually make marijuana itself illegal, it became very difficult to have anything to do with the drug without breaking the law in some way. Drug companies soon stopped using marijuana in medicines.

The public's attitude toward marijuana remained negative throughout the 1940s and 1950s. In the 1960s, however, that attitude began to change. Young people who wanted to rebel against the values and beliefs of their parents and other adults began to use the drug more openly and more often. Television news programs showed celebrities and hippies (usually young people who rejected the ideas of established society) smoking marijuana without any real consequences.

In popular music, songs like Brewer and Shipley's "One Toke Over the Line" and the New Riders of the Purple Sage's "Panama Red" celebrated the use of marijuana. In comedy acts and movies such as *Up in Smoke,* performers like Cheech Marin and Tommy Chong made people who smoked pot seem funny. In 1977, even President Jimmy Carter and his wife, Rosalynn, declared that possessing small amounts of marijuana should not be considered a crime. While scientists knew a great deal about the damage that "hard" drugs such as LSD and heroin did to the human body, they still didn't know very much about the physical and psychological effects of marijuana.

In the 1980s, the U.S. government toughened its position on illegal drug use. President Ronald Reagan and his wife, Nancy, launched a "war on drugs," a hard-hitting public awareness campaign. The government also instituted tougher criminal penalties for selling or using illegal drugs of all kinds, including marijuana. During the Reagan Administration (1981–88), marijuana use steadily declined.

Unfortunately, marijuana is once again growing in popularity among young people. In Chapter Four, we'll look at some of the reasons why. It's important to realize that today we know much more about the dangers of using marijuana than we did in the 1960s and 1970s. In the next chapter, we'll examine the harmful effects that marijuana can have on your brain and body.

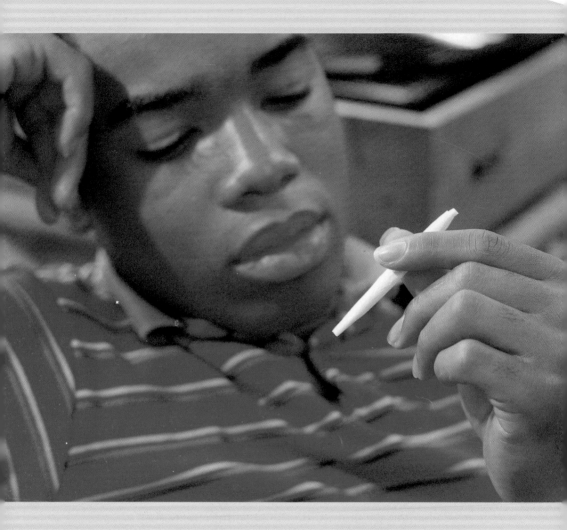

Thinking about trying marijuana? Read this chapter to find out what it does to your brain and body. You'll probably change your mind!

WHAT DOES MARIJUANA DO TO ME?

Today, we have enough information about the physical and mental effects of marijuana to realize that this drug can be dangerous. Adolescents are especially vulnerable to many of the health problems associated with marijuana because their bodies, minds, and spirits are rapidly developing. Marijuana impairs the brain's ability to learn and remember information. It interferes with thinking, problem solving, decision-making, and concentrating—the very skills you need most while your body and mind are still changing.

Marijuana also affects coordination, alertness, and the ability to perform even simple tasks. Driving a car while high, for example, greatly increases your chances of being involved in an accident. In a booklet called *Marijuana: Facts for Teens,* published by the National Institutes of Health, a study of people who visited emergency rooms after traffic accidents revealed that 15 percent of patients who had been driving a car or motorcycle had been smoking marijuana. Another 17 percent had both THC and alcohol in their blood. In Memphis, Tennessee, researchers found that 33 percent of 150 drivers arrested for recklessness showed signs of marijuana use, and 12 percent tested positive for both marijuana and cocaine. The bottom line: marijuana and driving do not mix. Nor is marijuana the harmless, relaxing drug that many kids think it is.

A More Potent Drug

The cannabis plant is a complex and unpredictable drug factory. THC, the main mind-altering chemical in cannabis, is a powerful **hallucinogen**—a substance that makes users perceive images or sounds that do not really exist. The amount of THC present in cannabis varies depending on the weather and soil conditions where it is grown. It can even vary from plant to plant.

Marijuana that is available to drug users today is much more potent than that of the 1960s and 1970s. The level of THC in plants grown 30 years ago was usually between 0.25 and 1 percent. Cannabis plants harvested in the United States today have THC levels that frequently exceed 20 percent. This increased potency not only makes marijuana more intoxicating, but it also increases the mental and physical health risks to those who use it.

What Does a High Feel Like?

The effects of using marijuana vary from person to person. They also depend on a number of outside factors, including:

- How potent the marijuana is (how much THC it contains)
- What the user is expecting to experience when he or she uses the drug
- The place where the drug is used (at a friend's house or at a concert, for example)
- How the drug is taken (whether it is smoked or eaten)
- Whether the user is also drinking alcohol or using other drugs

The most common sensation after using marijuana is a relaxed or euphoric feeling. A person who is high sometimes feels that ordinary sights, sounds, and tastes seem more intense. Time seems to pass very slowly. Sometimes users shift between moments of hysterical laughter and thoughtful silence. About a half hour or more after using marijuana, a person usually becomes drowsy and may even fall asleep.

Marijuana users also experience noticeable physical changes. They may become thirsty or extremely hungry—a condition often called "**the munchies.**" Their bodies respond to marijuana in other ways as well: blood pressure and heart rate increase, and eyes become bloodshot or red as the tiny vessels in them expand.

Every high is not pleasurable or relaxing, however. It is accurate to say that marijuana *intensifies* (strengthens) the physical and mental state the user was already in, rather than enhances (improves) it. New or inexperienced users of marijuana may be overcome by a sudden feeling of anxiety or paranoia. Other emotions—anger, fear, rejection, and hatred—may also be magnified.

Did You Know?

A recent study of 1,023 patients who were admitted to a hospital's shock trauma unit (which receives only the most seriously injured accident victims) found that one-third had detectable levels of marijuana in their blood.

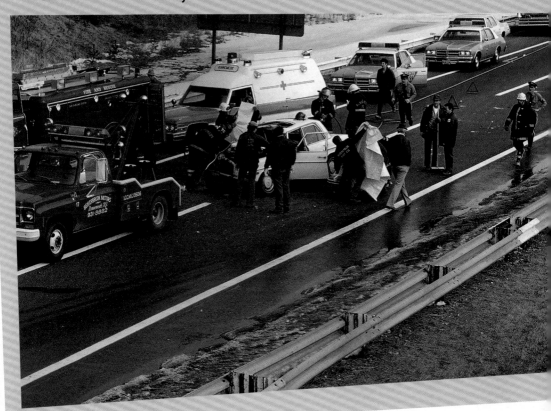

These feelings become even more intense when the marijuana is very potent or has been laced with other drugs. Under these conditions, users are also in danger of experiencing other adverse reactions, such as nausea, tremors, and fainting.

How Does Marijuana Affect My Health?

So far, research findings show a link between regular use of marijuana and a number of health problems that affect the respiratory, immune, and reproductive systems. Smoking marijuana may also increase your risk of developing cancer. Most important, marijuana affects your brain—it impairs your ability to learn, and it can cause short-term memory problems.

Marijuana and Your Brain

Marijuana causes some parts of the brain—such as those that control emotions, memory, judgment, and coordination—to lose balance and control. The chemicals in marijuana, especially THC, change the way a person sees, hears, smells, tastes, and feels things.

When someone uses marijuana, these chemicals travel through the bloodstream and quickly attach to special areas on the brain's nerve cells, called **neurons.** These areas are called **receptors,** because they receive information from other neurons and from chemicals. When a receptor receives information, it causes changes in the neuron.

The chemical in marijuana with the strongest impact on the brain is THC. Scientists recently discov-

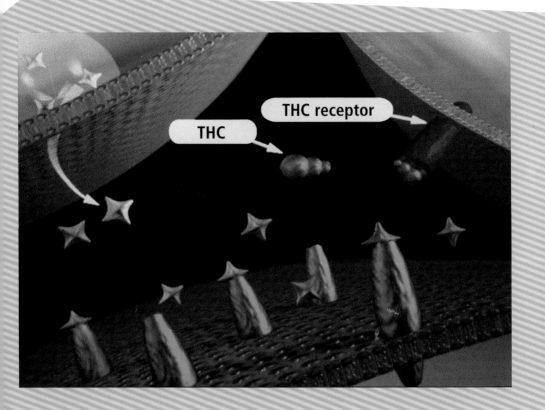

THC

THC receptor

This diagram shows a close-up of a synapse (the space between nerve endings) in the brain. Molecules of THC (the chemical in marijuana with the strongest effect on the brain) attach themselves to THC receptors (red) on the ends of neurons. The process is similar to the way neurotransmitters such as dopamine (shown here in orange) attach to their own receptors (blue).

ered that some areas of the brain have many THC receptors, while others have very few or none. These clues are helping researchers figure out exactly how THC works in the brain.

One region of the brain that contains a lot of THC receptors is called the **hippocampus.** The hippocampus

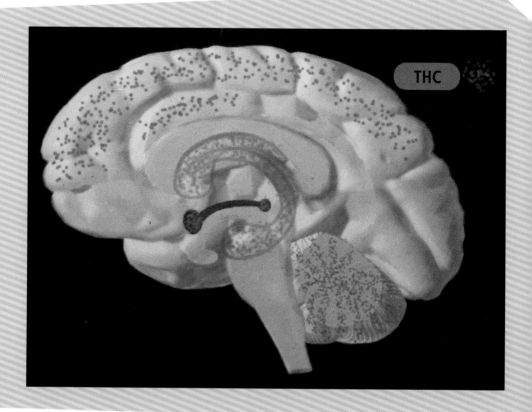

THC

The pink dots in this drawing show the regions of the brain that are affected by THC in marijuana and hashish. Notice that some of the dots are in the hippocampus (located under the solid purple section) and others are in the cerebellum (the lower right). Marijuana also affects the areas that control movement, sensation, and judgment.

processes memory, and when THC attaches to receptors in that part of the brain, it weakens short-term memory. The hippocampus also communicates with other parts of the brain that process new information into long-term memory. (Long-term memory allows you to remember today's math lesson or a new friend's phone number.)

When the brain is under the influence of marijuana, new information may not register and may be lost from memory forever.

The hippocampus is part of a larger region of the brain called the **limbic system.** Maybe you've heard about how marijuana can make some people giggle uncontrollably one minute and then feel paranoid the next. That's because THC influences the limbic system, which is responsible for emotions. Another area of the brain that is affected by marijuana is the **cerebellum,** which controls coordination and allows a person to perform tasks like playing a musical instrument, participating in a sport, or driving a car. This is why someone who is high on marijuana may be clumsy or uncoordinated.

Marijuana also has another kind of negative effect on the brain. Using it over a long period may cause what experts call **amotivational syndrome.** The user becomes unconcerned about the future, feels unambitious and apathetic, and becomes less physically active. For example, kids your age may lose interest in their favorite activities or sports, or they may stop doing their homework or attending classes regularly.

Did You Know?

A person who smokes five joints per week may be inhaling as many cancer-causing chemicals as someone who smokes 20 cigarettes—a full pack—every week. Marijuana users may also develop many of the same respiratory problems that tobacco smokers have, including chronic bronchitis and inflamed sinuses.

Marijuana and Cancer

Scientists are not sure whether regular marijuana smoking causes cancer. However, they do know that the smoke from a joint or bong has some of the same **carcinogenic** (cancer-causing) chemicals as tobacco smoke. One such chemical, benzopyrene, is present in both marijuana and tobacco smoke but is more concentrated in marijuana. Studies have shown that someone who smokes five joints a week may be inhaling as many harmful chemicals as a person who smokes an entire pack of cigarettes during the same period.

Marijuana's Effects on Your Respiratory System

People who smoke marijuana on a regular basis often develop the same kinds of breathing problems that cigarette smokers do. Both kinds of smokers experience frequent coughing, increased production of phlegm, wheezing, and recurring chest colds. Long-term exposure to marijuana smoke can also damage or destroy lung tissue, just as tobacco smoke can.

Recently, researchers compared the health of 450 daily marijuana smokers who did not use tobacco with another group who didn't smoke at all. They discovered that the marijuana smokers used more sick days and made more doctor visits than the group who never smoked.

Marijuana's Effects on Your Immune System

Your immune system fights infection and protects your body from bacteria and other harmful agents. The most powerful elements of the immune system are the white blood cells called **T lymphocytes** or **T cells,** which help the body resist viruses and fight cancer. Studies have shown that using marijuana weakens T cells, leaving them less able to fight disease.

Marijuana's Effects on Your Reproductive System

Using marijuana frequently or heavily can affect both male and female hormones. In men and boys, the drug lowers the level of **testosterone,** which triggers hair and beard growth, muscle mass development, and voice change. Marijuana use may even delay the onset of puberty in preteens.

In women and girls, heavy marijuana use can actually increase testosterone levels. Increased testosterone produces more body and facial hair and can cause or worsen acne in women and girls. Although it may be hard to imagine yourself as a parent, marijuana can affect that possibility, too. In boys, regular marijuana use can lower the sperm count (the number of sperm your body produces). In girls, it can interfere with the menstrual cycle. This means that male and female users of marijuana may have difficulty fathering or bearing children when they grow up.

Marijuana and Pregnancy

For some time, doctors have advised pregnant women to avoid drugs, alcohol, and many medicines because they can harm the fetus. Marijuana is no exception. Studies show that mothers who smoke marijuana while pregnant have babies that are shorter, weigh less, and have smaller heads than babies born to women who don't use the drug. And because smaller babies are often weaker, they run a greater risk of developing health problems. Doctors do not know whether babies born to mothers who smoked marijuana during pregnancy will have a higher risk of health problems as they grow up.

What Else Is at Stake?

Statistics show that people who smoke marijuana are also more likely to smoke cigarettes and drink alcohol. Using these "gateway drugs" puts users at greater risk of moving on to more powerful and addictive drugs such as cocaine and heroin. In an article addressed to adults entitled "It's Our Kids Who Are at Stake," the National Center on Addiction and Substance Abuse at Columbia University lists these facts:

- A 12- to 17-year-old who smokes cigarettes is 19 times more likely to use cocaine than one who does not smoke.
- An adolescent who drinks alcohol is 50 times more likely to use cocaine than one who does not drink.
- A 12- to 17-year-old who smokes pot is 85 times more likely to use cocaine than one who does not use pot.

- Adolescents who drink and smoke pot and cigarettes are 266 times more likely to use cocaine than those who don't use any of these gateway drugs.
- The earlier in life people use gateway drugs, the more likely they are to go on to harder drugs. Sixty percent of kids who begin smoking pot before the age of 15 will eventually use cocaine.

Another fact to keep in mind is that the body can develop a **tolerance** for marijuana and many other illegal drugs. This means that a user needs more and more of it to get the same kind of high he or she once got with a smaller amount. It is also possible to become dependent on marijuana—that is, to feel that it improves your daily functioning and that you need it to feel good. About 100,000 people each year seek treatment to help them stop using marijuana.

A person who is high on pot is also more likely to make foolish mistakes or to behave in an embarrassing way. One of the worst things about marijuana is that you can't always tell that your judgment is impaired. You may *think* that you can do things just as well as when you're not high, but it's not true.

Using poor judgment while under the influence of marijuana can endanger your life or the lives of your friends and family. "Marijuana makes you stupid," claims one teenager who used to smoke it. Knowing what the drug does to your brain, you can easily see what he means.

By now, you are probably wondering, "If marijuana

is so harmful, why do so many people use it?" The answer to this question is not an easy one. In the next chapter, we'll examine why some people choose to get involved with this drug.

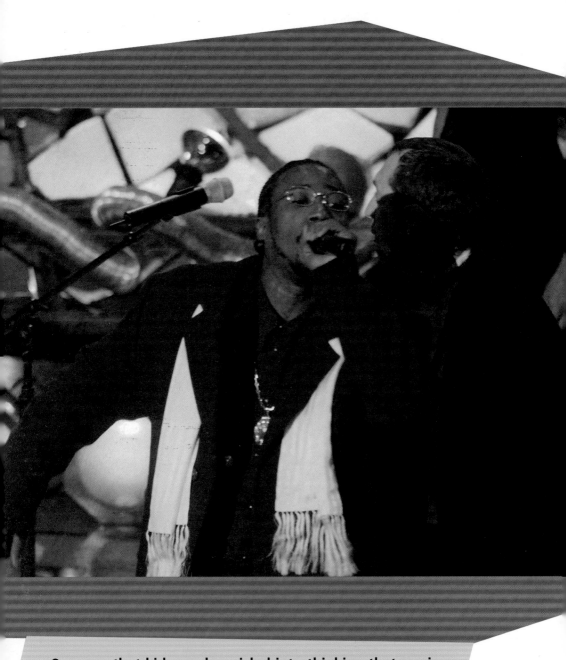

One way that kids can be misled into thinking that marijuana is "cool" is through music. Just as your parents or grandparents may have listened to songs that featured lyrics about drugs, you may hear a similar message from popular entertainers such as Wu-Tang Clan.

WHY DO PEOPLE USE MARIJUANA?

To find out why marijuana is still a popular drug, we must examine the reasons why people decide to start using drugs of any kind. We must also look at the ways in which outside influences convince people that smoking marijuana is fun, cool, or okay. Once we examine these facts, it will be easier to understand why some people decide to use marijuana despite all the risks.

Why Do People Use Drugs?

We all know what it feels like to want to belong to a social group. No one wants to feel disliked or left out when a friend is having a party or a group of kids is going to a concert, for example. But what happens when someone in the group does something you don't agree with or don't want to do? What if, on the way to the concert, one of your friends pulls out a joint? Even if you don't want to smoke pot, everyone else seems to be doing it. You don't want them to think you're a nerd by refusing. What do you do?

The feeling you experience when you're in a situation like this is called **peer pressure.** A peer—a friend, a sibling, or someone else of your own age group—does or says something to make you feel as though you have to act like them to fit in.

Sometimes, peer pressure is easy to spot. A person might come right out and say something to make you feel bad. "Come on, don't be a baby," your friend might say, or "Everyone else is doing it." Even if your friends don't say anything specific, you may still worry that they won't like you if you don't go along with them.

Peer pressure is one of the main reasons why kids begin to use drugs like marijuana. Even adults feel peer pressure, but when you're still growing up and trying to figure out exactly where you fit in, that pressure can be much stronger. After all, your friends are important to you. You sometimes feel more comfortable around them than you do with members of your own family. Often, they're facing the same struggles at school and at home that you are. That's why even if you don't want to try drugs, you might be tempted to take a drink of alcohol or a puff of marijuana to feel closer to them. In Chapter Five, we'll examine some of the ways you can conquer peer pressure and protect your health by refusing drugs.

Pressure from friends or relatives isn't the only reason kids start using drugs. Here are some of the other

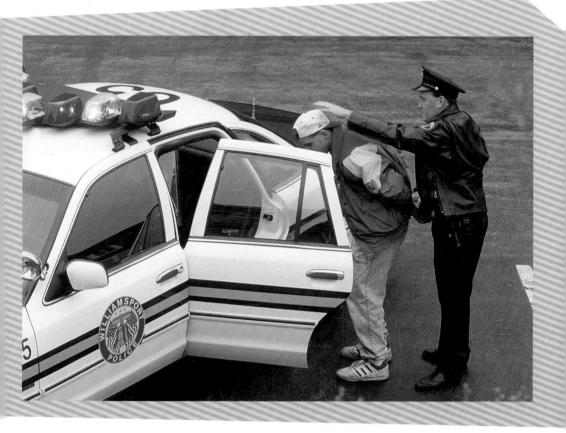

Whatever else you hear about marijuana, remember this: it's illegal. Depending on where you are caught, you can face heavy fines and be jailed for using, buying, or selling it.

reasons young people have given:

- To have fun or relax
- To feel more grown up
- Out of curiosity
- Because it seems exciting or rebellious
- To stop feeling lonely or depressed

Nothing is wrong with having any of these emotions or desires. Everyone feels them at one time or another—

especially when they're young. What's important is that you try to find ways to satisfy your sense of adventure or curiosity, or to help yourself feel less lonely or sad, in ways that are healthier than using drugs.

If you have already tried marijuana or other drugs, you have probably discovered that they *can* make you feel better. For a short time, maybe you can even forget about that bad grade you got in school or the fight you had with your brother. But in the long run, drugs won't solve your troubles or make your life more exciting. Nor will using drugs make you more grown up. In fact, now that you know the facts about marijuana, you have probably realized that drugs will only make your problems worse and make you seem less responsible and mature. Often, drug use even creates new problems.

Why Do People Use Marijuana?

Of all the illegal drugs in North America—cocaine, crack, heroin, LSD, PCP, amphetamines—marijuana is viewed as the least harmful. But as we have seen in earlier chapters, the fact that marijuana doesn't kill people directly does not make it harmless. And the damage done by marijuana can be just as serious as that caused by other drugs. Consider these facts:

- Between 1993 and 1994, more than one-fifth of all hospital emergency room episodes in the United States were related to marijuana or hashish use.
- In 1995, 54 percent of juveniles arrested for a criminal offense in Washington, D.C., tested positive for

marijuana. That same year, 41 percent of males (of all ages) arrested for criminal offenses in Chicago, Illinois, tested positive for marijuana. A similar statistic (42 percent) was found in Omaha, Nebraska. And in Canada, about 50 percent of the drug offenses recorded in 1995 were for possession of cannabis.

- In a 1993 study in Toronto, Canada, 92 percent of those found guilty of possessing marijuana were still using the drug a year later.

Why do some people view marijuana as less harmful than other drugs, or as not harmful at all? One of the reasons has to do with the way people have viewed marijuana throughout history, which we discussed in Chapter Two. Another reason is the way in which marijuana has been portrayed in advertising, song lyrics, movies, and television shows.

Not until the early 1980s did news stories, editorials, and TV specials began to focus on the problems caused by marijuana and other illegal drugs in the United States. TV and movie producers either began to avoid portraying drug use in their work or were careful to show its negative aspects. Many popular musicians of the 1980s also spoke out against drug use. As a result, during this decade the number of people aged 18 to 25 who reported using marijuana gradually began to fall.

One of the ways in which people began to learn more about drug abuse was through organizations like the Partnership for a Drug-Free America. The Partnership, which was formed in 1986, is a group of volunteers from

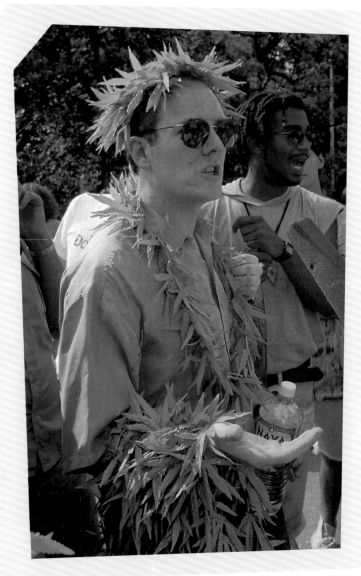

Wearing strands of marijuana leaves, Gregory Porter, the head of the National Organization to Reform Marijuana Laws (NORML), speaks to a crowd during a 1992 demonstration in New York City. Groups like NORML believe that marijuana should be made legal because of its medical uses.

the advertising, television, moviemaking, and publishing fields. Their main goal is to make sure that people are well-informed about what drugs can do to your brain and body. The group does this by producing advertisements that describe exactly what can happen to you when you smoke marijuana or use other drugs. If you read magazines, listen to the radio, or watch TV, you have probably seen or heard at least one of these ads.

Unfortunately, even though most kids your age don't smoke pot, the number of those who do has gone up in the 1990s. Researchers say that one of the main reasons more kids are smoking pot today is that a whole new generation of youngsters is finding out about the drug. They point out that kids your age weren't around in the late 1970s and early 1980s to hear about the dangers of using marijuana.

But this isn't the only reason. You, your friends, and your brothers and sisters have probably heard that there's nothing wrong with using marijuana. Nearly every day, you may get this message from the movies you watch, the CDs or tapes you listen to, or the baseball caps and T-shirts you see in the mall or at concerts. Maybe you've even come across websites on the Internet that promote marijuana as a cool or mellow drug that helps you to relax.

But think of this: these messages are just a different kind of peer pressure. The people who make the movies, videos, CDs, and clothing that celebrate marijuana are making money. They're counting on the fact that you'll want to fit in with your friends. You don't have to agree with them or buy their products to be popular.

Does Marijuana Still Have Medical Uses?

Not everyone believes that marijuana should be out-lawed. Some people think that growing, selling, and using it should be legal, in the same way that alcohol and cigarettes are. They want the U.S. government either to **decriminalize** (relax restrictions on) marijuana, or to **deregulate** it (make it legal again).

One of the biggest supporters of decriminalizing marijuana is a group called the National Organization for the Reform of Marijuana Laws (NORML), which was formed in 1970. That same year, the U.S. government passed a law called the **Controlled Substances Act** and named marijuana as a **Schedule I drug.** Marijuana fits in the Schedule I category because it meets three conditions:

- It has a high potential for abuse.
- It has no accepted medical uses.
- It is unsafe to use, even under the care of a doctor.

The members of NORML disagree with this ruling. They say that the cannabis plant has several medical uses, and that those who can benefit from its healing properties should not be denied the right to use it. They believe that we need to conduct more research on the good qualities of the drug. They also want marijuana to become a **Schedule II** drug, which would mean that physicians could legally prescribe it to certain patients.

Eventually, the U.S. Food and Drug Administration (FDA) approved of marijuana as a medicine that could be used only in very special cases. For example, patients who have AIDS often experience a rapid loss of weight, called "wasting." Some AIDS patients are able to fight the wasting by smoking marijuana or taking it in pill form, which improves the appetite.

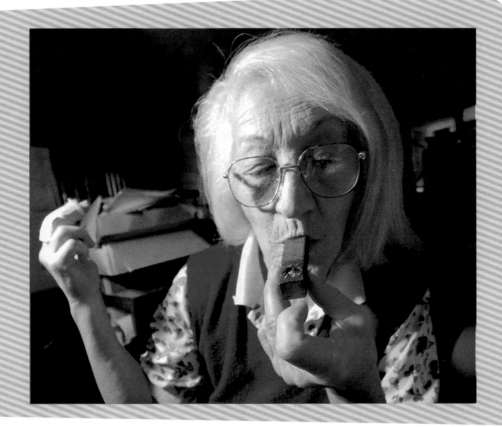

Compassionate use laws allow certain people to use marijuana as a medical treatment. Here, a woman who suffers from an eye condition similar to glaucoma puffs on a pipe filled with marijuana.

The cannabis plant has also been used by people undergoing a kind of cancer treatment called chemotherapy. In this treatment, a patient receives a mix of powerful medicines that kills cancer cells but that can also leave the patient nauseated. Scientists have discovered that THC, the chemical compound in marijuana that causes the "high," can help reduce nausea in cancer patients and help them to maintain their weight. Since

1985, THC has been available in a capsule called **Marinol** or **dronabinol.**

In the 1970s, some researchers also discovered that marijuana seemed to help patients who have **glaucoma,** an eye disease in which the pressure of the fluid within the eyeball becomes too great. Marijuana helps to reduce the pressure and lower the patients' risk of permanent eye damage.

In 1996, two U.S. states—Arizona and California—became the first to pass laws making it legal for patients and physicians to use, grow, or possess marijuana only for the purpose of medical treatment. These permitted exceptions are called **compassionate use laws.** Between 1978 and 1996, 34 states and the District of Columbia passed laws that *recognize* marijuana's medical value (25 of these laws are still in effect today), but these states' laws do not make marijuana legal. In the rest of the country, marijuana is illegal without exception.

Many people are opposed to compassionate use laws. They fear that it is easy to abuse such laws because a physician only has to "recommend," not "prescribe," marijuana. They also point out that Arizona's law is dangerous because it allows physicians to recommend other Schedule I drugs, such as LSD and heroin.

If Marijuana Can Help People, Why Is It Illegal?

Now you know about the ways in which marijuana might help people with specific ailments. You know about special exceptions that allow certain people to use marijuana lawfully. You may start thinking that a substance that helps sick people can't really hurt you.

But make no mistake: marijuana is not a harmless drug. Even legal substances that you buy at the supermarket or drugstore, such as cold medicines and pain relievers, can be extremely harmful if used improperly. These medicines are prepared and packaged under strict regulations that control their quality, strength, and safety. An illegal drug like marijuana is not subject to these restrictions, so you never know how powerful or dangerous a particular dose may be. Nor will you know whether the joint your friends are urging you to try has been laced with an even more addictive and dangerous substance, such as PCP. Even in patients who are allowed to use marijuana for medical reasons, the drug can have serious side effects and cause other health problems.

Using marijuana even once can have long-lasting effects on your mind and body. Using it more than once may increase your risk of cancer. It can affect your ability to remember things and solve problems. It might also affect your chances of having children someday. It may even cause permanent brain damage.

If you haven't tried marijuana, you're not alone. Many high schoolers graduate without having used it even once. If you have tried marijuana, and if you're having a hard time staying away from it, there are many things you can do to stop using it and become a healthy, drug-free person.

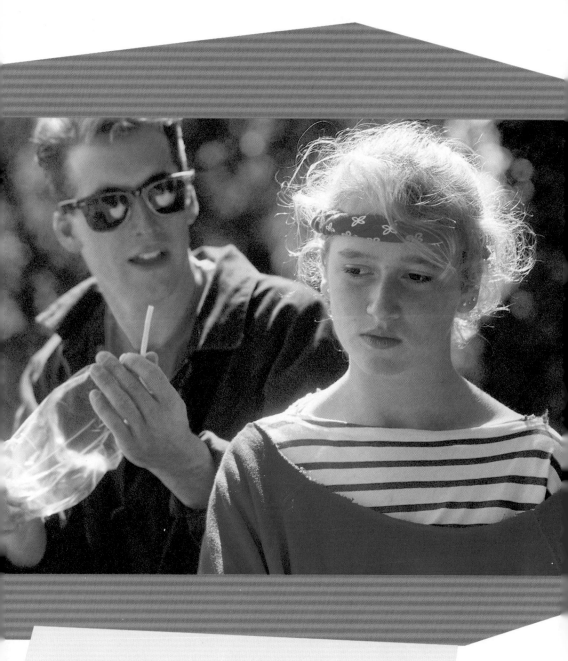

If someone offers you marijuana, how do you turn it down? Read this chapter for some ideas.

5

YOU CAN MAKE A DIFFERENCE

N ow that you know about the harmful effects of marijuana and other gateway drugs like cigarettes and alcohol, you need to know how to protect yourself and your friends. In this chapter, we will learn how you can say no to peer pressure and stay drug-free. We'll look at some of the ways you can recognize the signs that you or someone you know may be abusing marijuana or other drugs. Finally, we'll find out where you can get help for your friends, your relatives, or yourself.

How Do I Say No Without Losing My Friends?

It's tough to stand out from the crowd. The desire to fit in can be a very powerful feeling. But you don't *have* to give in to peer pressure. There are ways to avoid doing

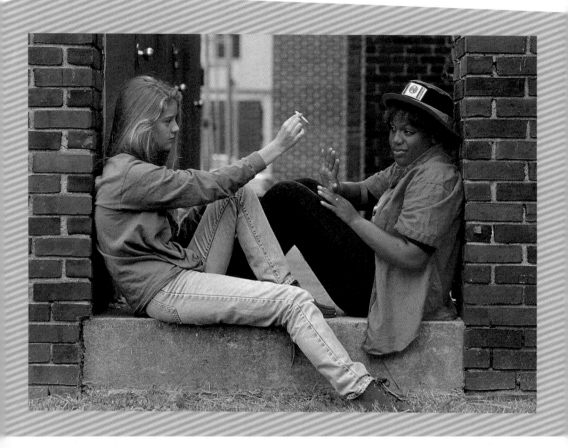

Even if you don't want to use marijuana, you may feel pressured by your friends to try it. Remembering how marijuana affects your mind and body may help you to say "No, thanks."

things you don't want to do while still feeling like part of the gang. Remember that group of your friends on the way to a concert? Chances are, you're not the only one in the group who doesn't want to smoke pot. Others may feel the same way, but they may also be afraid to speak up. But if you want to do what's best for you, you have to stand up for yourself.

This isn't always easy, of course. It takes courage. You fear that you'll lose your friends. But you may find that if you do say no, other friends who may have been afraid to speak up will take your side because they'll know they are not alone. And it's often easier than you might think to say "No, thanks."

Here are a few other ways that you can take control of your life and resist drugs:

- Skip parties or activities where you know there will be alcohol or other drugs.
- Hang out with friends who don't use drugs.
- Find new after-school activities. Check with recreation centers, youth clubs, libraries, or other local organizations to see whether they offer tutoring, sports, music lessons, or craft classes.
- Get involved in drug-free activities like dances, movies, community service projects, or walk-a-thons. Ask your friends to join you.
- Organize a drug awareness program for your school, church, or community center.

What Are the Signs That Someone Is Using Marijuana?

One of the reasons some kids and adults end up using pot regularly is that they can "get away with it." It is often hard to tell when someone is high on marijuana. When used alone, without alcohol, marijuana doesn't always make you seem especially loud or giggly, or make you unsteady on your feet.

But there are a few signs you can watch for. The most obvious one is redness of the eyes. This happens because marijuana increases the heart rate and makes the tiny blood vessels in the eyes dilate (expand). The user may also act silly or giggle for no reason, or may seem dizzy and have trouble walking. Another sign is extreme sleepiness or hunger ("the munchies"). You may notice a sweet, burnt scent on the person's clothing or in the air. Someone who uses marijuana may frequently carry eyedrops or own drug paraphernalia such as pipes or rolling papers (used to make joints).

How Can I Tell If Someone I Know Has a Problem with Drugs?

As we have seen, marijuana is a gateway drug. Using it may lead to "harder" or more addictive drugs, like cocaine or crack. It's not always easy to tell whether a friend or relative has been abusing drugs. Most people don't want to tell someone close to them that they have a problem. They may even try to hide or deny it. But you can look for certain signs that someone you know may be struggling with a drug or alcohol problem. Here are some of them:

- Getting high on drugs or getting drunk on a regular basis
- Lying about the amount of alcohol or other drugs they're using
- Avoiding you or other friends in order to get high or drunk

- Giving up activities such as sports, homework, or hanging out with friends who don't drink or use other drugs
- Having to use increasing amounts of marijuana or other drugs to get the same effect
- Constantly talking about drinking or doing other drugs
- Pressuring other people to drink alcohol or use other drugs
- Believing that they need to drink or use other drugs to have fun
- Getting into trouble with the law or getting suspended from school for an alcohol- or other drug-related incident
- Taking risks, including sexual risks and driving under the influence of alcohol or other drugs
- Feeling tired, run-down, hopeless, depressed, or even suicidal
- Missing work or school, or performing tasks poorly because of drinking or other drug use

Keep in mind that some of these signs, such as changes in mood or behavior, poor job or school performance, and depression, might be signs of other problems. They could also be symptoms of an illness that you may not know about. Be sure to talk to an adult you trust or one who is trained to recognize alcohol and other drug abuse. A doctor, nurse, priest, rabbi, minister, counselor, scout leader, coach, or parent can give you advice about what to do next.

How Can I Tell If I Have a Problem with Drugs?

Drug and alcohol problems affect all kinds of people, regardless of age, sex, race, marital status, income level, or way of life. If you abuse drugs and think you're not like others who do, you're wrong. Just like anyone else who abuses drugs, you can seriously endanger your body and mind—or even your life. To find out whether you have a problem, try to answer the following questions honestly:

- Can I predict the next time I will get drunk or use other drugs?
- Do I think that I need alcohol or other drugs to have fun?
- Do I turn to alcohol or other drugs to make myself feel better after an argument or confrontation?
- Do I have to drink more or take more drugs to get the same effect I once felt with a smaller amount?
- Do I drink or use other drugs when I'm alone?
- When I drink or use other drugs, do I forget certain segments of time?
- Am I having trouble at work or school because of alcohol or other drug use?
- Do I make promises to others or to myself to stop drinking or using other drugs, but then break them?
- Do I feel alone, scared, miserable, or depressed?

If you answered "yes" to any of the above questions, you may have a drug problem. Don't be discouraged,

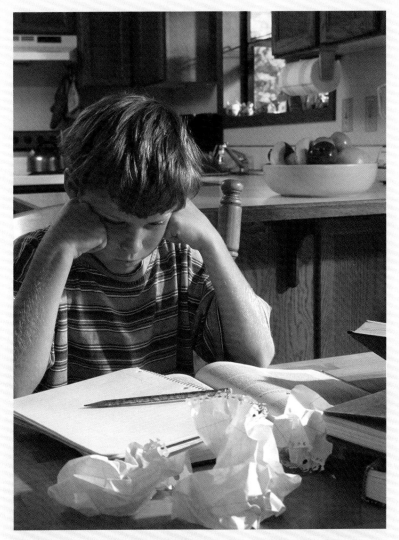

Rather than solving problems, drugs like marijuana can cause new ones, including difficulty concentrating or performing schoolwork.

though. You are not alone. Millions of people around the world have triumphed over drug abuse and are now living healthy, drug-free lives.

Where Do I Go for Help?

No matter where you live, you can find help for drug problems from numerous national, state, and local organizations, treatment centers, referral centers, and hotlines. Some treatment services and centers require their patients to remain at the center as **inpatients** for several weeks or months. Others provide **outpatient** counseling, meaning that you attend scheduled therapy sessions but return home after each treatment.

A number of resources are listed in the back of this book. Some of the resources you may find in your community are:

- Drug hotlines
- Treatment centers
- City or local health departments
- Local branches of Alcoholics Anonymous, Al-Anon/Alateen, or Narcotics Anonymous
- Hospitals or emergency health clinics

Maybe you are hesitant or fearful about seeking help. Most drug treatment programs provide group (or family) therapy for people with alcohol or other drug problems, so you will not have to face your troubles alone. All you have to do is pick up the phone and take that first step. The trained and experienced people on the other end of the line will take it from there.

Try to keep this in mind as well: research shows that when drug abusers get appropriate treatment—and when they follow the prescribed program—*treatment*

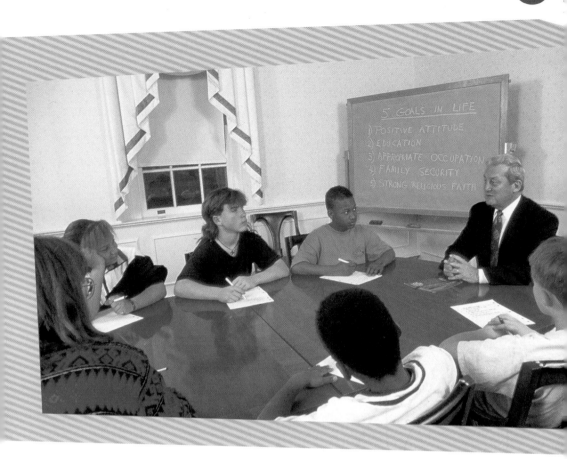

One of the most important elements of drug abuse treatment is psychological counseling. Former drug users may see a counselor privately or meet with others in a group session, like the one shown here.

can work. Getting treatment will not only help you conquer your drug problem, but it will also give you the skills and the strength that you need to avoid using drugs in the future. Being healthy and drug-free is the best way to make sure that you grow up to achieve your dreams.

amotivational syndrome—a loss of motivation in an individual that is accompanied by apathy, lack of concern for the future, and diminished physical activity. Some researchers believe that marijuana may cause amotivational syndrome in users.

blunt—a marijuana-filled cigar.

bong—a large pipe used to smoke marijuana.

Cannabis sativa—the scientific name of the plant that is the source of marijuana and hashish.

carcinogenic—causing or contributing to the growth of cancer.

cerebellum—the part of the brain that controls coordination.

compassionate use laws—U.S. state regulations that allow physicians and patients to use marijuana legally to treat illnesses such as glaucoma, nausea from cancer treatment, and weight loss in AIDS patients.

Controlled Substances Act—a law passed in 1970 that organized drugs into five categories, called Schedules, that regulate their use in the United States.

decriminalize—to relax legal restrictions. A decriminalized substance is still regulated by certain laws; a deregulated substance has no legal restrictions on it.

delta-9 tetrahydrocannabinol—*see* **THC.**

deregulate—to make legal again. A deregulated substance has no legal restrictions on it; a decriminalized substance is still regulated by certain laws.

dronabinol—a medicine formulated from THC, one of the chemical compounds in the cannabis plant. Dronabinol helps combat nausea in cancer patients and helps AIDS patients maintain their weight. *See also* **Marinol.**

gateway drug—a relatively weak drug whose use may lead to experimentation with stronger drugs like cocaine and heroin.

glaucoma—an eye disease marked by increased pressure of the fluid in the eyeball; it can lead to eye damage or loss of vision.

grass—a common nickname for marijuana.

hallucinogen—a substance that causes the user to perceive objects or visions that are not real, or distorts the user's perception of objects or events.

hashish, hashish oil—a drug made from the resin of the *Cannabis sativa* plant.

hemp—another name for the *Cannabis sativa* plant, the source of marijuana, hashish, and THC.

heroin—the name given to diacetylmorphine, one of the strongest of the opiate drugs.

hippocampus—the part of the brain responsible for processing memory.

inpatient treatment—a drug rehabilitation program in which a person stays at, or is checked into, the clinic or hospital where the treatment will take place.

joint—one of the most common names for a marijuana cigarette.

lace—to add a substance to; marijuana is often laced with dangerous drugs such as PCP.

limbic system—the region of the brain that controls emotions.

LSD—lysergic acid diethylamide, a hallucinogenic (mind-altering) drug synthesized from a fungus that grows on the rye plant.

Marinol—the manufacturer's name for dronabinol, a medicine formulated from THC, one of the chemical compounds in the cannabis plant. Marinol helps combat nausea in cancer patients and helps AIDS patients maintain their weight. *See also* **dronabinol.**

(the) munchies—a nickname describing the increased feeling of hunger induced by smoking marijuana.

neurons—nerve cells.

outpatient treatment—a drug rehabilitation program in which a person lives at home and attends scheduled therapy and education sessions.

paraphernalia—apparatus like pipes or roach clips used with illegal drugs.

PCP—phencyclidine, sometimes called "angel dust"; an animal tranquilizer that is often mixed with marijuana. PCP is extremely dangerous; even one use can cause serious mental illness.

peer pressure—words or actions by a friend, a sibling, or someone else of your own age group that make you feel as though you have to act like them to fit in with the group.

psychoactive—affecting the mind or behavior.

receptor site—a special area of a cell that combines with a chemical substance to alter the cell's function.

recreational—intended to be refreshing or to provide a diversion.

resin—a yellowish or brownish substance that oozes from certain trees and plants. Some resins are used in making varnishes, lacquers, plastics, and many other products. Hashish and hashish oil are products of the resin from the cannabis plant.

retting—the process of separating hemp fibers from the cannabis plant.

roach clip—a device for holding a marijuana cigarette.

Schedule I drug—a drug that is considered unsafe to use, has no known medical value, and has a high potential for abuse. Marijuana, LSD, and heroin are Schedule I drugs.

Schedule II drug—a drug that has a high potential for abuse but has proven medical value. Morphine, amphetamines, and codeine are Schedule II drugs.

sinsemilla—a potent, seedless form of marijuana made from the unfertilized female cannabis plant.

speedballing—injecting a mixture of cocaine and heroin.

taint—to contaminate or mix with another substance; marijuana is often tainted with chemicals or dangerous drugs such as PCP.

T cell or **T lymphocyte**—a special type of white blood cell that helps the human body fight infection and disease.

testosterone—a male sex hormone. Research shows that heavy use of marijuana may decrease the level of this hormone in males and increase it in females.

THC—an abbreviation for delta-9 tetrahydrocannabinol, the chemical found in cannabis that is most responsible for the high users get from marijuana.

tolerance—the need to increase the dosage of a drug in order to get the same result that was previously achieved by using smaller amounts.

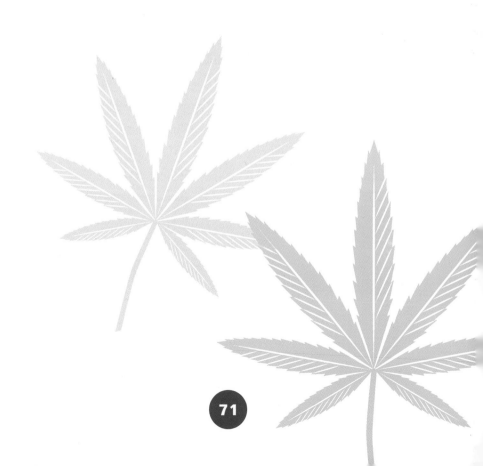

BIBLIOGRAPHY

Connolly, Beth. *Through a Glass Darkly: The Psychological Effects of Marijuana and Hashish.* Philadelphia: Chelsea House Publishers, 1999.

Croft, Jennifer. *Drugs and the Legalization Debate.* New York: Rosen Publishing Group, 1997.

Kuhn, Cynthia, Scott Swartzwelder, and Wilkie Wilson. *Buzzed: The Straight Facts About the Most Used and Abused Drugs From Alcohol to Ecstasy.* New York: W. W. Norton and Company, 1998.

Myers, Arthur. *Drugs and Peer Pressure.* New York: Rosen Publishing Group, Inc., 1995.

National Clearinghouse for Alcohol and Drug Information, Center for Substance Abuse Prevention. *Drugs of Abuse.* NCADI Publication No. RP0926. Rockville, MD: National Clearinghouse, 1998.

National Institute on Drug Abuse. *The Brain's Response to Marijuana* (Mind Over Matter series). NIH Publication No. 97-3859. Rockville, MD: National Institute on Drug Abuse, 1997.

———. *Marijuana: Facts for Teens.* NIH Publication No. 95-4037. Rockville, MD: National Institute on Drug Abuse, 1995.

———. *Marijuana: Facts Parents Need to Know.* NIH Publication No. 95-4036. Rockville, MD: National Institute on Drug Abuse, 1995.

———. *What Can Parents Do?* Videotape. NCADI Stock #VHS82. Washington, DC: U.S. Department of Health and Human Services, 1995.

Oliver, Marilyn Tower. *Drugs: Should They Be Legalized?* Springfield, NJ: Enslow Publishers, 1996.

Schleichert, Elizabeth. *Marijuana.* Springfield, NJ: Enslow Publishers, 1996.

FIND OUT MORE ABOUT MARIJUANA AND DRUG ABUSE

The following list includes agencies, organizations, and websites that provide information about marijuana and other drugs. You can also find out where to go for help with a drug problem.

Many national organizations have local chapters listed in your phone directory. Look under "Drug Abuse and Addiction" to find resources in your area.

Agencies and Organizations in the United States

American Council for Drug Education
164 West 74th Street
New York, NY 10023
212-758-8060
800-488-DRUG (3784)
http://www.acde.org/
wlittlefield@phoenixhouse.org

Center for Substance Abuse Treatment / Information and Treatment Referral Hotline
11426-28 Rockville Pike, Suite 410
Rockville, MD 20852
800-622-HELP (4357)

Girl Power!
U.S. Department of Health and Human Services Office on Women's Health
11426 Rockville Pike, Suite 100
Rockville, MD 20852
800-729-6686
http://www.health.org/gpower
gpower@health.org

Just Say No International
2000 Franklin Street, Suite 400
Oakland, CA 94612
800-258-2766

Marijuana Anonymous World Services
P.O. Box 2912
Van Nuys, CA 91404
800-766-6779
http://www.marijuana-anonymous.org/
MAWS98@aol.com

Narcotics Anonymous (NA)
P.O. Box 9999
Van Nuys, CA 91409
818-773-9999

National Center on Addiction and Substance Abuse at Columbia University
152 West 57th Street, 12th Floor
New York, NY 10019-3310
212-841-5200 or 212-956-8020
http://www.casacolumbia.org/home.htm

National Clearinghouse for Alcohol and Drug Information (NCADI)

P.O. Box 2345
Rockville, MD 20847-2345
800-729-6686
Fax: 301-468-6433
800-487-4889 TDD
800-HI-WALLY (449-2559, Children's Line)
http://www.health.org/

National Council on Alcoholism and Drug Dependence, Inc. (NCADD)

12 West 21st St., 7th Floor
New York, NY 10017
212-206-6770
800-NCA-CALL (622-2255)
http://www.ncadd.org/

National Family Partnership

1159B South Towne Square
St. Louis, MO 63123
314-845-1933

Office of National Drug Control Policy

750 17th Street, N.W., Eighth Floor
Washington, DC 20503
http://www.whitehousedrugpolicy.gov/
ondcp@ncjrs.org
888-395-NDCP (6327)

Parents Resource Institute for Drug Education (PRIDE)

3610 Dekalb Technology Parkway, Ste 105
Atlanta, GA 30340
770-458-9900
Fax: 770-458-5030
http://www.prideusa.org/

Agencies and Organizations in Canada

Addictions Foundation of Manitoba

1031 Portage Avenue
Winnipeg, Manitoba R3G 0R8
204-944-6277
Fax: 204-728-0225
http://www.mbnet.mb.
    ca/crm/health/afm.html

Addiction Research Foundation (ARF)

33 Russell Street
Toronto, Ontario M5S 2S1
416-595-6100
800-463-6273 in Ontario

Alberta Alcohol and Drug Abuse Commission

10909 Jasper Avenue, 6th Floor
Edmonton, Alberta T5J 3M9
http://www.gov.ab.ca/aadac/

British Columbia Prevention Resource Centre

96 East Broadway, Suite 211
Vancouver, British Columbia V5T 1V6
604-874-8452
Fax: 604-874-9348
800-663-1880 (BC only)

Canadian Centre on Substance Abuse

75 Albert Street, Suite 300
Ottawa, Ontario K1P 5E7
613-235-4048
Fax: 613-235-8101
http://www.ccsa.ca/

Ontario Healthy Communities Central Office

180 Dundas Street West, Suite 1900
Toronto, Ontario M5G 1Z8
416-408-4841
Fax: 416-408-4843
http://www.opc.on.ca/ohcc/

Saskatchewan Health Resource Centre

Saskatchewan Health, T.C. Douglas Building
3475 Albert Street
Regina, Saskatchewan S4S 6X6
306-787-3090
Fax: 306-787-3823

Websites

Avery Smartcat's Facts & Research on Children Facing Drugs

http://www.averysmartcat.com/druginfo.htm

D.A.R.E. (Drug Abuse Resistance Education) for Kids

http://www.dare-america.com/index2.htm

Elks Drug Awareness Resource Center

http://www.elks.org/drugs/

Hazelden Foundation

http://www.hazelden.org/

Join Together Online (Substance Abuse)

http://www.jointogether.org/sa/

National Institute on Drug Abuse (NIDA)

http://www.nida.nih.gov

Partnership for a Drug-Free America

http://www.drugfreeamerica.org/

Reality Check

http://www.health.org/reality/

Safe & Drug-Free Schools Program

http://inet.ed.gov/offices/OESE/SDFS

U.S. Department of Justice Kids' Page

http://www.usdoj.gov/kidspage/

YOU CAN'T AFFORD IT

Despite what you may have heard,
selling illegal drugs will not make you rich.

In 1998, two professors, Steven Levitt from the University of Chicago and Sudhir Venkatesh from Harvard University, released a study of how drug gangs make and distribute money. To get accurate information, Venkatesh actually lived with a drug gang in a midwestern city.

You may be surprised to find out that the average street dealer makes just about $3 an hour. You'd make more money working at McDonald's! Still think drug-dealing is a cool way to make money? What other after-school jobs carry the risk of going to prison or dying in the street from a gunshot wound?

Drug-dealing is illegal, and it kills people. If you're thinking of selling drugs or you know someone who is, ask yourself this question: is $3 an hour worth dying for or being imprisoned?

WHAT A DRUG GANG MAKES IN A MONTH*

	During a Gang War	No Gang War
INCOME (money coming in)	$ 44,500	$ 58,900
Other income (including dues and blackmail money)	10,000	18,000
TOTAL INCOME	**$ 54,500**	**$ 76,900**
EXPENSES (money paid out)		
Cost of drugs sold	$ 11,300	$ 12,800
Wages for officers and street pushers	25,600	37,600
Weapons	3,000	1,600
Tributes (fees) paid to central gang	5,800	5,900
Funeral expenses	2,300	800
Other expenses	8,000	3,400
TOTAL EXPENSES	**$ 56,000**	**$ 62,100**
TOTAL INCOME	$ 54,500	$ 76,900
MINUS TOTAL EXPENSES	- 56,000	- 62,100
TOTAL AMOUNT OF PROFIT IN ONE MONTH	**- 1,500**	**14,800**

* adapted from "Greedy Bosses," *Forbes*, August 24, 1998, p. 53.
Source: Levitt and Venkatesh.

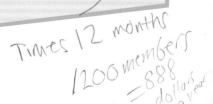

Times 12 months
1200 members
=888
dollars
a year

INDEX

PICTURE CREDITS

page
6:   Courtesy Office of National
     Drug Control Policy, the
     White House
12: Richard Hutchings/Photo
     Researchers, Inc.
17: AP/Wide World Photos
19: Photofest
22: James King-Holmes/Photo
     Researchers, Inc.
27: Photofest
32: Richard Hutchings/Photo
     Researchers, Inc.
36: Andrea Krause/Photo
     Researchers, Inc.
38: National Institute on Drug
     Abuse
39: National Institute on Drug
     Abuse
46: AP/Wide World Photos
49: © 1994 Terry Wild Studio
52: AP/Wide World Photo
55: AP/Wide World Photo
58: Richard Hutchings/Photo
     Researchers, Inc.
60: Richard Hutchings/Photo
     Researchers, Inc.
65: PhotoDisc Vol. 24, #24045
67: Bachman/Photo
     Researchers, Inc.

JUDY L. HASDAY, a native of Philadelphia, Pennsylvania, received her B.A. in communications and her Ed.M. in instructional technologies from Temple University. A multimedia professional, she has had her photographs published in several magazines and books, including a number of Chelsea House titles. She is also a freelance author of biographies for young adults, including *James Earl Jones* and *Madeleine Albright.*

THERESE DE ANGELIS received an M.A. in English Literature from Villanova University. She was the contributing editor for Chelsea House's *The Black Muslims, Rosie O'Donnell,* and the WOMEN WRITERS OF ENGLISH series. She is also the author of several books for young adults, including *Native Americans and the Spanish* in the INDIANS OF NORTH AMERICA series and *Louis Farrakhan* in the BLACK AMERICANS OF ACHIEVEMENT series.

BARRY R. McCAFFREY is Director of the Office of National Drug Control Policy (ONDCP) at the White House and a member of President Bill Clinton's cabinet. Before taking this job, General McCaffrey was an officer in the U.S. Army. He led the famous "left hook" maneuver of Operation Desert Storm that helped the United States win the Persian Gulf War.

STEVEN L. JAFFE, M.D., received his psychiatry training at Harvard University and the Massachusetts Mental Health Center and his child psychiatry training at Emory University. He has been editor of the *Newsletter of the American Academy of Child and Adolescent Psychiatry* and chairman of the Continuing Education Committee of the Georgia Psychiatric Physicians' Association. Dr. Jaffe is professor of child and adolescent psychiatry at Emory University. He is also clinical professor of psychiatry at Morehouse School of Medicine, and the director of Adolescent Substance Abuse Programs at Charter Peachford Hospital in Atlanta, Georgia.